# Eat Foods That Grow

## A simple mantra for growing your energy

Kathryn Peterson
www.kamakatyoga.com

# Overview

Eat foods that grow
and you will grow too...

I mean growing your energy,
raising your vibrational frequency.

The cells in our body create an electromagnetic field that travels by waves. Our vibrational frequency refers to how fast these waves move.

Greater vibrational frequencies mean
greater power, passion, pleasure.

Plants are the foods with the highest vibrational frequencies. Fruits, vegetables, nuts, seeds, olives.

My name is Kat and I am a private yoga teacher.
Eating foods that grow is how I learned to feel at peace with eating. No restrictions, no cycling, no stress.

Eating foods that grow is how I help many of my clients to overcome and reverse diabetes, high blood pressure, impotency, fatigue, depression.

Eating foods that grow,
raising our vibrational frequency,
makes it easier for us to harness our sexual energy,
makes it easier for us to transform lust into love.

Many of my clients think that plant-based eating will make them lose protein. But actually, plant-based eating gives us sufficient and superior protein. I have never had a protein deficient client. Most Americans consume nearly double the recommended amount of protein. Deficiency is statistically nonexistent.

Many of my clients think that plant-based eating will make them gain weight. But actually, plant-based eating makes it easier for us to lose weight. I have never had a client become obese from eating too many fruits. Most of my clients become obese from eating too many processed foods. Fast food, soda, chips, cereals, vegetable oil, meats.

Many of my clients think that plant-based eating will make their life more complicated. But actually, plant-based eating makes your life more simple…

You don't have to read any labels.
You don't have to count any calories.
You don't have to limit how many plants you eat.

Less is more…
Less processing of the food means
more energy in the food.

You simply eat foods that grow.

# Mantra

A mantra is a word or phrase that
focuses our mind on our intention.

It can be easy for the mind to be taken over by thoughts…
Remembering all those messages, meetings, promises made
to those closest to you. Forgetting what your mind, your
body, your spirit needs along the way.

When we are stressed, when we are lost in our thoughts,
it can be easy to eat food without any awareness.

When we let ourselves be taken over by processed food
we let ourselves be taken over by stress, fatigue, dis-ease.

A mantra is a tool for becoming aware,
anchoring us in the midst of a thought storm.

When it comes time to eat. Whether you are moved by a
business lunch, a break in your schedule, a growl of your
stomach. It can be easy to take over your health with high
vibrational foods. It can be easy to eat mindfully.

It can be easy to simply practice the mantra…

Eat foods that grow.

Eat foods that grow.

Eat foods that grow.

Eat foods that grow.

Eat foods that grow.

Eat foods that grow.

Eat foods that grow.

Eat foods that grow.

Eat foods that grow.

Eat foods that grow.

Eat foods that grow.

Eat foods that grow.

# Wabi-sabi

A Japanese legend tells of Rikyu, whose tea master asked him to clean the yard. After raking and weeding the space to perfect orderliness, he shook the cherry tree until blossoms dripped onto the ground.

That is wabi-sabi…
the beauty of imperfection,
the beauty of impermanence.

Many of my clients ask me for help with plant-based eating. I simply tell them to eat more fruits and vegetables. Eat more foods that grow.

And I say this can be done in a wabi-sabi way.

You don't need to eat the same foods every day.
You don't need to eat the same meals every day.
You don't need to eat the same times every day.

Just simply eat as many fruits and vegetables as you can.

It doesn't have to look like a preconceived notion of balance. You can eat four bananas, three carrots, and an avocado. You can eat two pounds of grapes. You can eat salad with pineapple and peanut butter.

Just simply eat foods that grow.

# Breakfast

Eat foods that grow for breakfast.

Wake up with a burst of nutrients in your mouth…
Bananas, berries, grapes, apples, pears, melons.
Mango, pineapple, papaya, coconut.

You can make a simple oatmeal with oats and hot water.
Adding cinnamon, spices, seeds.
And as much fresh fruit as you can!

You can make a simple toast with nut butter.
And as much fresh fruit as you can!

You can have eggs with spinach, tomato, mushrooms.
And as much fresh fruit as you can!

Soon your body will become trained to crave
he nutrients, the high vibrations of fresh fruits
first thing in the morning.

Try any wabi-sabi combination to
eat foods that grow…

# Salad

Eat foods that grow in a salad.

The simplest tip that I tell my clients who want to lose weight, is to eat a large salad before your regular meal. Because you are filling up with the nutrients of foods that grow, you will eat less of your regular meal. You will feel full, you will feel high vibrational without sacrificing.

Make your salad with only foods that grow…

Lettuce, spinach, arugula, kale.
Tomato, carrots, peppers, cucumber.
Garbanzo beans, kidney beans, edamame.
Mushrooms, olives, onions, artichokes, beets.
Sunflower seeds, pumpkin seeds, pine nuts, walnuts.

Try dressing your salad with balsamic vinegar, apple cider vinegar, olive oil. Try to avoid industrial salad dressing that typically contains processed oils and processed chemicals.

Try ordering your dressing on the side if you are ordering out. This way you can minimize the amount of processed oils that might be coming your way.

Try any wabi-sabi combination to
eat foods that grow…

# Roasting

Eat foods that grow with the oven.

Simply set your oven to 400 degrees Fahrenheit.
Chop up vegetables and place them on a large pan.
Add olive oil and all the spices that you like.
Let them roast for about 45-60 minutes.

Try roasting different combinations of…
Potatoes, sweet potatoes, zucchini, eggplant.
Broccoli, green beans, brussel sprouts.
Peppers, onions, mushrooms.
Tofu, peas, garbanzo beans.

Try any wabi-sabi combination to
eat foods that grow…

# Steaming

Eat foods that grow in a rice cooker,
an amazing tool that requires hardly any effort.

Simply add equal parts rice and water to the cooker.
Then add vegetables in the steaming tray.
Set it and forget it until it pops.

Try steaming different combinations of…
Broccoli, cabbage, carrots, cauliflower, corn.
Peppers, onions, spinach, green beans.

Try adding avocado or tahini on top.

Try any wabi-sabi combination to
eat foods that grow…

# Snacking

Eat foods that grow for snacks.

Carry simple foods that are easy to eat on the go.

Try simple fruits that come in a peel.
Bananas, mandarin oranges, grapefruit.
You don't even need to wash them!

Try miniature versions of fruits and vegetables.
Persian cucumbers, cherry tomatoes, baby carrots.
You don't even need to cut them!

Try foods that you can wash and take.
Apples, pears, berries, grapes.
Sliced celery, sliced zucchini.

Try simple dips for your fruits and vegetables.
Nut butter, tahini, hummus, guacamole.

Try raw nuts and seeds.
Pumpkin seeds, sunflower seeds,
Almond, walnuts, peanuts.

When you go to the corner store for a snack, look for
foods that grow. Bananas and unsalted peanuts.

Try any wabi-sabi combination to
eat foods that grow…

# Restaurants

Eat foods that grow at restaurants.

Try eating from the appetizers…
Vegetable soup, lentil soup, miso soup.
Edamame, shishito peppers, vegetable spring rolls.
Hummus, baba ganoush, mixed olives.

Try eating from the sides…
Rice and beans, plantains, guacamole.
Sautéed vegetables, roast vegetables, roast potatoes.

Try eating from the salads…
Papaya salad, bean salad, seaweed salad.
Green salad, beet salad, mushroom salad.
Remember to order the dressing on the side.

Try eating entrees that have the most foods that grow…
Vegetable curry, lentil curry.
Vegetable pasta, vegetable pizza.
Sauteed tofu, grilled seitan, black bean burger.
Dishes that come with beans, greens, vegetables.

Try any wabi-sabi combination to
eat foods that grow…

# Eating Foods That Grow:
# Guided Practice

**Eat foods that grow…**

Every morning I make oatmeal for breakfast with oats, cinnamon, ground flax. Adding in the sweet flavors of fruits like juicy pears and ripe bananas.

Keeping my energy high with foods that grow…
Keeping my snackpile stocked with bananas, mandarin oranges, blueberries, raw peanuts.

A bursting salad with kale, cucumber, tomato, alfalfa, carrots, corn, red grapes, avocado, apple cider vinegar. And then the black beans and rice from the night before.

My energy keeps growing with those foods that grow…
Snacking on bananas and bananas for days…

A simple dinner with chopped potatoes, broccoli, onions, and tofu. All roasted together on a pan in the oven with olive oil and seasonings.

And in that perfect time of year, a dripping slice or watermelon makes you taste like the nectar of gods…

**Eat foods that grow with a full schedule…**

Breakfast is oats and an apple
because that's the only fruit I find.

I stop at the store while I'm on my way to teach yoga.
Greek yogurt, banana, oranges for a snack.

Then after teaching, I grab a bagel and coffee.
Oops! And also, yum! Eat foods that grow…
I order it with peanut butter and have another orange.

For lunch I cook the leftover lentil soup from last night's
dinner. I add the leftover rice from last night's dinner.
I add some spinach that I find in the refrigerator.

Some more oranges for an early evening snack.

For dinner, I go out and have a delicious salad.
I order it with no cheese, and the dressing on the side.
I share a dish of wild halibut, navy beans, leeks.

And a very special, all-natural dessert at home…

**Eat foods that grow with a tight wallet…**

Morning breakfast with oats, cinnamon, fruit.

100% peanut butter with banana can work on a sandwich
for breakfast, snack, lunch. You can even add alfalfa sprouts
for a cheap burst of nutrients.

Leftover rice and lentils for lunch. Cook with water and
spices. You can add frozen kale of spinach for a cheap burst
of nutrients. Fresh greens when the price is right.

You can cook rice, lentils, seasonings in one big pot
that lasts for days and costs just a few dollars…

Look for the deals and let them dominate…

When potatoes and sweet potatoes and bursting out the
ground. When it's fall in New York and apples are selling
for less than a dollar per pound.

When it's tropical and the mangoes are dripping from
every tree… you can eat 10 mangos a day for free!

Buying frozen and seasonal food is
a budget friendly way for
eating foods that grow.

**Eat foods that grow with a carnivore…**

You know that oatmeal and fruit is my favorite breakfast…
Try adding berries, bananas, seeds to yogurt.
Try adding onion, spinach, tomato, mushroom to eggs.

If you order a breakfast sandwich, order fruit to go with it.
Eat the fruit first for filling up with those nutrients…

If you order a sandwich for lunch, order salad to go with it.
Eat the salad first for filling up with those nutrients…
Remember to order your salad with foods that grow only.
Remember to order the dressing on the side.

If you order anything else, order salad to go with it.
Eat the salad first for filling up with those nutrients…
Remember to order your salad with foods that grow only.
Remember to order the dressing on the side.

Try adding roasted or sauteed vegetables to meat dishes.
Try adding roasted or sauteed vegetables to pastas.
Try adding arugula, sprouts, greens to anything.

Remember that plant-based doesn't mean plants only.

Simply eat more and more foods that grow…

# Thank You

Thank you for reading this guide.

Remember that the whole is greater than the sum of its parts. The whole of you is more than skin, bones, organs. The whole of an apple is more than vitamins, calories, fiber. This is what is meant by whole foods eating. Simply eating the whole food that grows.

Eating foods that grow is a simple way for growing our energy, our blood flow, our vibrational frequencies.

Plant-based eating helps us stay healthy when it comes to our weight, our blood pressure, our hormones, our libido.

Thank you for practicing mindfulness when it comes to eating foods that grow…

One simple mantra revitalizing your mind, body, spirit.

If you have any questions about eating foods that grow. If you would like to learn more about my work…

www.kamakatyoga.com